I0504686

FREEZING YOUR WAY TO HEALTH

Facts and Misconceptions Regarding Ice Baths

Anthony S. Willis

Disclaimer

Copyright by Anthony S. Willis, 2023. All rights reserved.

Before this document is duplicated or reproduced, the publisher's consent must be gained. Therefore, the contents cannot be stored electronically, transferred, or in a database. Neither in Part nor complete can the document be copied, scanned, faxed, or retained without approval from the publisher or creator

TABLE OF CONTENTS

INTRODUCTION

Ice baths are becoming increasingly popular in sports treatment and recovery. Still, this popularity has also given rise to several myths and raised many concerns regarding the risks involved and the efficacy of the treatment.

A wellness craze like ice baths makes people genuinely desire to know up front whether it works because it appears so painful. Athletes often employ this toe-numbing procedure to ease muscle discomfort. It has been hailed via social media by celebrities such as Lady Gaga, Kim Kardashian, Harry Styles, Kendall Jenner, Lizzo, Madonna, and Harry Styles.

These appear to be fantastic testimonials; however, we are all mindful that celebrities are not health professionals. We will thus go through all the information you require on ice baths, including what they do, all the information you need to decide, and how to use them properly.

How does taking an ice bath affect the body?

Ice baths, as the phrase implies, include briefly immersing the body in cold water. Ice baths — or "cold water immersions," Therapy with cold water, chilly therapies, or cold plunging— aren't new, but their recognition has fluctuated in the past few years; what exactly transpires within one's body when on an ice bath is quite simple. It said that when you apply ice or cold to a spot, your blood vessels tighten, and less blood flows to that location. Therefore, if it affects your complete body, you will experience contraction of those blood vessels all over, with an emphasis on your arms and legs to keep most of your heat away from your core region.

Blood does not flow as fast to such locations when blood arteries contract. In general, decreased blood flow means less inflammation - at least briefly. While some advice 10 to 15 minutes, 2 to 10 minutes for a beginner, as it is always recommended to start small.

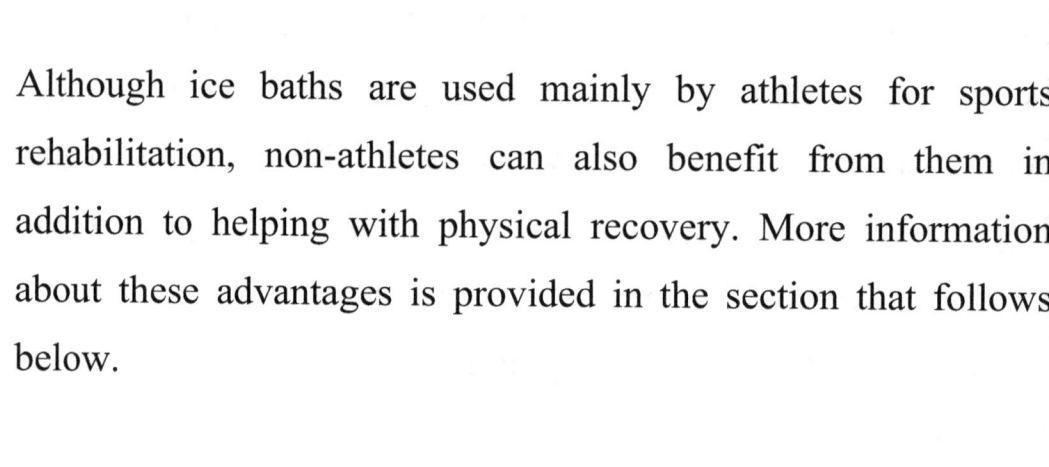

Although ice baths are used mainly by athletes for sports rehabilitation, non-athletes can also benefit from them in addition to helping with physical recovery. More information about these advantages is provided in the section that follows below.

The Advantages of Taking Ice Baths

Ice baths are well-known for their numerous health benefits that can help practically everyone on their health path. Plunging is an excellent addition to your regimen for general health and wellness, benefiting your mind and body. Some advantages are as follows: Creatine kinase, an enzyme secreted into the circulation after muscle cells are injured during strenuous exercise, also showed promising results, according to scientists.

Evidence suggests that taking an ice bath after engaging in a strenuous activity may be beneficial. Still, there are also psychological and practical benefits to cold water immersion.

❖ Taking an ice bath can help reduce swelling and pain. It can suppress pain receptors and reduce inflammation, almost like a natural sedative. Individuals who suffer from inflammatory illnesses such as rheumatoid arthritis might find that immersion in cold water helps minimize swelling or discomfort caused by outbreaks or after workouts.

❖ Using them helps you relax and rest more soundly. After a strenuous workout, you might find that immersing yourself in cold water helps you feel more relaxed. "After getting extremely hot and incredibly sweaty,

To summarize, you can anticipate the following advantages:

❖ **General Health:**

    ✓ Support for the immune system,

    ✓ improved blood flow,

    ✓ accelerated metabolism,

    ✓ assistance with weight loss,

    ✓ and increased energy

❖ **Mental Health:**

    ✓ Improve mood;

    ✓ Develop self-control;

    ✓ Strengthen mental fortitude;

    ✓ Reduce stress;

    ✓ Boost energy;

    ✓ Lessen worry and despair

❖ **Healing & Pain Reduction**

    ✓ Reduced inflammation,

    ✓ lessened and prevented muscle soreness,

    ✓ improved performance,

✓ increased physical toughness,

✓ and decreased chronic pain.

❖ **the skin**

✓ Reduce eye puffiness,

✓ tighten skin,

✓ remove fine lines and wrinkles,

✓ and boost blood flow to give skin a healthy sheen.

Medically Supported Research on Ice Baths

In-depth research on cold immersion and ice baths has been conducted by the National Library of Medicine (NLM), and the results highlight several benefits supported by scientific studies.

Athletes that took ice baths after their workouts reported decreased muscular discomfort and could train for more extended periods after their ice baths, according to the findings of a study conducted by the NLM. Similarly, two investigations performed by other researchers, one in 2016 and the other in 2011, found that bikers experienced reduced soreness after immersing in cold water for ten minutes.

According to the findings of yet another NLM study, exposure to cold water produces an "immune stimulation" effect, which, in layman's terms, boosts your immunological system. Taking cold showers has been shown in several studies to improve one's immune response, as well as to reduce inflammation and feelings of anxiety. After a few weeks of hydrotherapy, the signs and symptoms of depression were shown to improve, according to a study found on Science Direct.

These are only some researches I thought was particularly noteworthy, although the complete list is far longer. This research section will continue to have new additions made to it as we come across additional reputable and pertinent sources of information, which will be shared with you in my subsequent books.

According to an article published by SSM Health, preliminary research indicates that persons who frequently indulge in ice baths have a lower risk of contracting infections caused by bacteria, which suggests that ice baths can help the body's immunological system.

According to the article, cold plunges and regular ice baths may enhance mood and help people adapt to stress over Time. Scientists believe the approach can generate a stress response that activates the neural system. This response may help people become more resilient to the effects of stress.

According to Breitbach, the best techniques for ice baths and cold-water submersions include water temperatures ranging from 50 to 55 degrees and soaking for approximately 15-20 minutes.

Ice baths and cold-water submersions should be avoided by people who are sensitive to cold and have particular health concerns, including high blood pressure and cardiovascular disorders, amongst others.

Because being in cold water for an extended period raises the danger of developing hypothermia, it is essential to keep track of the passing of Time and to be aware of any changes that may occur in the body.

Ice Bathing: Some Essential Facts

There are a few things you need to take into consideration before jumping into an ice bath to ensure that your experience is as joyful and beneficial as it can be.

• If you are susceptible to the cold or suffer from any other ailments, you should discuss the possibility of taking a cold plunge with your primary care provider first.

Take a quick shower to get emotionally and physically ready for the fight. You will better understand how your body will react to the cold on a more local level, which will help you better manage your reactions in the future.

Consider how well you can withstand the cold. It is acceptable to begin the process at approximately 60 degrees Fahrenheit and then gradually lower it. It is also good to start with a time limit of 30 seconds to one minute and gradually increase it to two or ten minutes.

• We recommend anywhere from two to ten minutes, but it's excellent, to begin with just one or two minutes as you become used to taking an ice bath.

Instructions on How to Get Ready for an Ice Bath

There is much more to ice baths than simply filling your bathtub with ice and water. Here are some other benefits of ice baths. It would be best if you got ready for your ice bath in advance by doing some preparation work so that the process goes as smoothly and delightful as possible. If this is your first Time taking an ice bath, there are a few things to remember.

Before you begin to construct an ice bath, check to be that you have all of the necessary components, including:

- If you want to make your ice bath, you'll need a tub or vessel, a thermometer, a bag (or two), and a hose if you use a stand-alone tub without a faucet.

Other things you should do to get ready:

- Before, during, and after your ice bath sessions, learn a few breathing methods you can use.
- Towels and dry clothes, like long-sleeved shirts, pants, and socks, should be kept nearby in case you need them after diving.
- Have your timer set and within reach of you at all times.

- Immediately change into your ice bath attire. You should at least wear shorts and a T-shirt, but some individuals also wear a sweatshirt, booties, and gloves. The minimum acceptable attire is **shorts and a T-shirt.** It is up to you to decide.

- Plan to get out of the ice bath gradually and engage in some light activity to warm up.

The Step-by-Step Guide to Taking an Ice Bath at Home

After completing the preparatory tasks outlined above, it is now Time to prepare your ice bath and enjoy it.

1. Fill a bathtub with ice and cold water, and continue adding ice until the water reaches the desired temperature.

After you have gathered your ingredients and post-ice bath attire (as described in the section above), fill your tub with cold water to the desired level, and then add ice one piece at a time until the temperature reaches a point where it is bearable. It is OK to begin somewhere between 55- and 60 degrees Fahrenheit and proceed later.

2. Get a timer and keep it where you can easily access it

Only two to three minutes of meditation per day is all it takes to get the advantages of this practice, but it's terrific. To begin with only one minute, I recommend anywhere between two and five minutes, but you're OK to go up to ten minutes.

3. Step into the Ice Bath, and begin counting the Time.

After warming up your lungs with some pre-plunge breathwork for a few minutes, start the timer on your watch, and then slowly enter the freezing water of your ice bath.

4. Let Your Mind and Body Soak While You Concentrate on Your Breathing Work. Concentrate your attention on something you have command over, such as your breathing, rather than the temperature of the water. By engaging in some form of breathwork, such as taking big breaths followed by a little pause before expelling, you can reduce the pace of your heartbeat, enhance your circulation, and make yourself feel more comfortable. Additionally, it will prevent you from concentrating on the icy water by diverting your attention to something else entirely.

5. Get Out of the Ice Bath and Get Some Light Exercise to Warm Up. When the alarm goes off, slowly leave the ice tub and pat yourself dry. While doing it, pat yourself on the back for being such a champion! After that, change into the clothing you would wear after the ice bath, and then think about performing some light activity to warm up, such as stretches or jumping jacks. If you want to have the most significant possible

experience with an ice bath and get relief from any problems you may be experiencing, don't forget also to consider the safety precautions that are listed below in the safety section.

Possible Limitations or Drawbacks

Ice bathing, like most other activities concerning one's health, presents a small but manageable number of potential dangers. Keeping the above safety advice and rules in mind will significantly lower the likelihood of experiencing any adverse effects. The following are some of the potential downsides:

Injuries caused by cold: If you remain in cold water for an extended period, you risk getting frostbite or hypothermia; however, you will most likely experience warning symptoms before either condition occurs. To prevent this from happening, make sure that the temperature of the water is only turned down as far as it is safe for you to do so, which should be between 39- and 60 degrees Fahrenheit. In addition, limit each session to between two and ten minutes.

Dizziness: This dizziness may be caused by the constriction of your blood vessels when you drink cold water. This is another excellent reason to select a water temperature suitable for you and limit the amount of Time you spend submerged to a few minutes during each session. If you feel lightheaded at any point during your Time in the ice bath, you should get out of there immediately.

Are there any dangers associated with taking ice baths?

Even though taking an ice bath is usually considered safe, only some should do it. "First and foremost, there are health issues where you must consult with your doctor before taking an ice bath because it can have unpleasant and possibly harmful effects, noting that this is due to how the cold water tightens the blood vessels. "Ice baths can have adverse and potentially dangerous consequences,

Heart disease, high blood pressure, diabetes, peripheral neuropathy, poor circulation, venous stasis, and cold agglutinin disease are some of the disorders that fall under this category.

If you have any concerns about taking an ice bath, discussing them with your primary care physician, even if you do not suffer from pre-existing diseases, is best. The use of ice baths by **children, particularly younger children**, should **be avoided**.

People also need to be careful not to utilize ice baths to numb the pain caused by a more severe injury. "If you had a fracture, or an injured ligament or tendon... and you're using this to push through the pain, that's a **big no-no,"**. You would need to see a sports medicine physician to get a proper diagnosis of the issue.

Common Misconceptions Regarding Ice Baths

Many myths and misunderstandings float around concerning ice baths, and almost all of them are entirely false. To provide you with an accurate picture of ice baths and dispel some rumors and misconceptions surrounding them, we will dispel some of those myths and stories below.

MYTH: Ice baths are only beneficial for athletes.

The use of ice baths is not restricted to athletes alone;

TRUTH: in fact, people who are not athletes can, do, and even ought to partake in them. People can take a cold plunge for a variety of health reasons in addition to physical recovery, including the following:

• to boost one's metabolism and immune system

• to build resilience and increase one's ability to manage stress

• better boost one's blood circulation over the long term

• to maintain one's mental health

MYTH: Immersing Yourself in Ice Water Will Give You a Cold or Dehydration

TRUTH: There is no proof that ice baths cause dehydration or colds, but you should still observe safety rules, just in case.

No evidence supports the claim that taking an ice bath or being exposed to cold water would cause you to acquire a cold.

As for hypothermia, provided that you adhere to the safety rules, there is very little probability that you will ever suffer from this condition. You would be able to detect the onset of hypothermia early on and have enough Time to get out of there before it became severe. If you are new to ice baths or have a low cold tolerance, it is recommended to start at roughly 55 to 59 degrees Fahrenheit and Plunge for two to five minutes the first time you do it to be on the safe side.

MYTH: I Can't Take an Ice Bath Because I Don't Have Time or I'm Too Busy

TRUTH: The recommended Time for a cold plunge is between two and five minutes, but you can survive in the water for as little as two minutes.

Consider the following: It will take you far less Time than watching your favorite show that is thirty minutes long, and it will be a more productive use of your Time than lazily scrolling through your feed for an hour.

If you still find yourself saying, "I'm too busy," think about the things you do daily and ask yourself whether or not those things are productive uses of your Time-tested or whether or not they are time wasters. At the very least, you should go for a cold plunge once or twice every week. You should discover a few minutes you do not use or are wasted. You can either have results or excuses, but not both; therefore, the question is: which will you choose?

The traditional process of preparing an ice bath can take some time because you have to go out and get ice, carry it inside, fill the container with water, add some ice, and then keep monitoring the water temperature until you have it just right. If you use the revolutionary tub known as the Ice Plunge, however, you may drastically cut down the amount of Time spent setting up your ice bath and start enjoying it much sooner. You may save a significant amount of Time by using the Plunge because all you have to do is set the desired temperature, and then you can have cold filtered water on demand.

MYTH: Ice Baths Are Too Expensive

TRUTH: The investment in your health pays off in the long run, and there are ice bathing options that won't break the bank.

Taking care of your health and maintaining a healthy lifestyle is an investment in your future. Although ice bath containers and tubs may appear expensive at first, you should consider purchasing one as an investment in the same way that you would consider buying a treadmill, weight room equipment, and other home fitness equipment.

Conclusion

You are now prepared to begin using ice baths, even if you are not an athlete or a cold-water therapy fan. Utilize an at-home ice bath to experience their many physical and psychological advantages for yourself, and always remember safety first.

www.ingramcontent.com/pod-product-compliance
Lightning Source LLC
Chambersburg PA
CBHW070914220526
45466CB00005B/2210